Hugo Barcia M.

PALLIATIVE USE OF INOTROPICS IN END-STAGE HEART FAILURE

Hugo Barcia M.

PALLIATIVE USE OF INOTROPICS IN END-STAGE HEART FAILURE

An approach beyond the usual

ScienciaScripts

This book is a translation from the original published under ISBN 978-620-2-25050-4.

Publisher:
Sciencia Scripts
is a trademark of
Dodo Books Indian Ocean Ltd. and OmniScriptum S.R.L Publishing group
Str. Armeneasca 28/1, office 1, Chisinau MD-2012, Republic of Moldova, Europe
Printed at: see last page
ISBN: 978-620-5-38763-4

DEDICATION.

I dedicate this work to God because he is the provider of all things, to my wife and my children who were a fundamental pillar to strengthen my life, who during times of adversity always remained firm and supported me, they have not allowed me to collapse but rather have managed to make me stronger, to my parents who gave me life and taught me the values that today define me as a person and professional since my childhood and even when I grew up they do not neglect my being. To my sister Mishel with her husband and my nephews and nieces; to Natalia who kept me trusting and waiting; to the Mendoza Solorzano family who gave me support and understood the effort we have made together.

The heart of the discerning acquires wisdom, and
the ear of the wise seeks knowledge.

Pr. 18:15

ACKNOWLEDGEMENTS.

To God for having accompanied and guided me throughout my career, for being my strength in moments of weakness and for giving me a life full of opportunities, experiences and perseverance. To my wife Elizabeth and my children Hugo, Efraín and Jeremías who have been part of the effort in building this foundation, to my parents Hugo and Beatriz who rejoice in the fruits of their lives overcoming difficulties, to my sisters Mishel and her husband Carlos, and Natalia who are allies of this path, my nephews Sophia, Carlos, Micaela and Kayla who are reasons for inspiration. And also a special thanks to the training team of the Universidad Abierta Interamericana, Thank you very much.

INDEX

SUMMARY

OBJECTIVE: The aim of this research was to systematically review the palliative use of inotropes in end-stage heart failure.

MATERIALS AND METHODS: This is a systematic study with a quantitative, descriptive, cross-sectional approach. We used scientific databases such as PubMed, Medline, Scopus, and Medes studies related to the use of inotropic drugs for palliative purposes in patients diagnosed with terminal heart failure. Systematic reviews and meta-analyses were included, taking into account that the intervention was carried out in patients with decompensation due to their own evolution of the disease.

RESULTS: The pooled studies included 336 adult patients with a mean age of 65 years, with no variability in race, sex and marital status. All studies assessed quality of life demonstrating improvement in NYHA functional class (decreasing on average 1.5 points). The 6-minute walk test increased by the same percentage as CF. Hospital admissions decreased by 50% since initiation of therapy.

In relation to complications, arrhythmias occurred in 34% of all patients analysed; it should be noted that not all studies included arrhythmias as complications within the study; these manifestations were assessed by activation of the ICD. Another complication was catheter-associated infection (central line) in 12% of treated patients. The studies evaluated a probability of survival with 36 patients yielding the following results: a median of 3.4 months overall, and with the Kaplan Meier survival curve were 3, 6, and 12 months corresponding to 51%, 26%, 6% of patients respectively, but this was not established as a relevant indicator due to the insufficient sample included in the review.

KEY WORDS: End-stage heart failure, palliative care, inotropics.

CHAPTER I

THEORETICAL APPROACH.

INTRODUCTION

According to the World Health Organisation (WHO), cardiovascular diseases are the leading cause of death worldwide in the last 20 years. Heart failure (HF) is a dynamically evolving disease with frequent flare-ups, which is complex to conceptualise[1] . On average 1% of the population over 40 years of age acquires an initial stage of HF and this percentage doubles every 10 years to 10% in those over 70 years of age[2-3] . This implies the great impact of the disease in terms of incidence and prevalence; HF currently affects more than 6 million adults in the United States, and 8 million patients are projected by 2030[4] .

Throughout the life of a heart failure patient it is often necessary to apply a series of complex and invasive treatments, which are less effective in advanced stages of the disease. [5]

The American College of Cardiology/American Heart Association (ACC/AHA) Guidelines address palliative inotropic therapy as part of an overall plan to improve quality of life.[7]

This review suggests that inotropic drugs would have a place as palliative treatment in this group of patients.

1. RESEARCH APPROACH.

The problem to be investigated was to analyse the different studies focusing on interventions on the use of inotropics as palliative therapy in patients with end-stage heart failure (HF), benefits and risks in terms of evidence.

The main research question was: Can Inotropics be used as palliative therapy in End-Stage Heart Failure ?

2.- OBJECTIVES

2.1.-Objective General

To investigate by systematic review the palliative use of inotropes in end-stage heart failure.

2.2.-Specific Objectives

To determine the benefits of palliative use of inotropes in end-stage heart failure.

Determine risks regarding the palliative use of inotropes in end-stage heart failure.

3.- THEORETICAL FRAMEWORK

3.1.- END-STAGE HEART FAILURE AND PALLIATIVE CARE.

Palliative care is defined by the World Health Organisation as an approach that improves the quality of life of patients and their families in the face of life-threatening illness by preventing and alleviating suffering through early identification, assessment and treatment of pain and other physical, psychosocial and spiritual problems[6] . During palliative care, conventional treatment is not withdrawn; a direct advantage is the therapeutic adjustments that will optimise symptom management.

According to the 2013 ACC / AHA guidelines, palliative care has a Class 1B recommendation and is effective for patients with end-stage heart failure; this group experiences stages of decompensation, followed by frequent improvement and stability[7] (fig.1), however, the emphasis on hospice is poor, and its application is less than 10% in total patients[5] .

3.2.- CRITERIA FOR THERAPEUTIC CHOICE.

The identification of the CTI patient is not far from the clinician who is able to use different tools and predictive models to determine a definitive decision.

Useful clinical criteria for predicting prognosis include worsening symptoms, recurrent hospitalisations, alterations in cardiopulmonary exercise testing, biomarkers, and predictive tools such as the Kansas City questionnaire for patients with chronic heart disease (fig. 2), thus offering a chance of hope for improved quality of life. It is therefore the responsibility of the specialist physician to integrate the above guidelines into the consultation to assess the patient's overall prognosis[8] .

3.3.- PALLIATIVE THERAPY WITH INOTROPICS IN STROKE.

The choice of patients for palliative inotropic therapy in end-stage disease should encompass assessments in the following aspects: psychological, clinical, and social, as well as non-candidates for advanced therapies such as cardiac transplantation and ventricular assist devices (table 1).

3.4.- CLINICAL FACTORS

Inotropic dependence marks an important starting point for the identification of the functional grade of CKD, in that patients receiving palliative inotropics must demonstrate improvement of symptoms; and worsening of symptoms with withdrawal. Analysis of the studies showed that the main reasons for stopping inotropic drug withdrawal were end-organ hypoperfusion, hypotension and renal dysfunction; in addition, conventional treatment including diuretics should be optimised[8] .

3.5.- EVIDENCE FOR INOTROPICS AS PALLIATIVE THERAPY

In recent decades, pharmacological strategies have been used to stabilise the clinical manifestations of heart failure and improve survival (fig. 3); however, they do not halt progression and result in high mortality in the final stage of HF[1] . In fact, the AHA/ACC consensus guidelines define stage D of HF as the terminal phase, a situation where the patient manifests a high symptomatic burden refractory to conventional treatments and without the option of transplantation or mechanical ventricular assistance; and it is at this point where inotropics have a proposed indication for chronic use, with direct and indirect relation to hospitalisation; This is carried out with the application of intermittent or continuous intravenous therapy for palliative purposes endorsed by the AHA/ACC in 2013 (recommendation IIb - Level of evidence B) and described as palliative treatment in patients with advanced HF who are not candidates for transplantation or circulatory assist devices[9] (Table 1).

Outpatient use of inotropes in patients with CCI has been analysed for approximately 20 years and success has depended on several factors, including the optimised regimen in conventional treatment, and the stability of symptoms at the start of inotropic treatment. It should be emphasised that the initiation of inotropic therapy is in a hospital setting, and an important factor for a successful transition to inotropics in an outpatient setting is a strong specialised home support system.

In 2003 a study was published by Ray Hershberger et al. where they implemented a programme for continuous outpatient inotropic support; where 36 post-discharge inotropic dependent patients, all with CTI criteria, were included in the programme; rehospitalisations were 46 in total; 6 subjects accounted for 24%; and 22% had at least 1 rehospitalisation; they analysed a median survival of 3.4 months; and Kaplan Meier survival at 3, 6 and 12 months was 51%, 26% and 6% respectively (fig. 3.1). Most patients died at home and chose not to undergo resuscitation attempts[10] .

While it is true that many clinical trials in the 1990s through 2000 demonstrated that the use of intravenous or oral inotropics in acute or chronic heart failure was consistently associated with decreased survival and/or increased risk of adverse cardiovascular events. In some of these studies, 6-month mortality exceeded 50%, however, these studies were not designed to address the use of inotropics as palliation (Figure 3.1).

Another group in the United States analysed the need to implement a palliative and hospice care programme for patients with end-stage heart failure; these patients received intermittent infusions of inotropic drugs, the study included 73 patients, 50% were eligible for the programme by inclusion criteria and their own decision, the drugs used were dobutamine with an initial dose of 2.5 mcg/kg/min and milrinone with an initial dose of 0.375 mcg/kg/min.375 mcg/kg/min, treatments were started on a two or three times a week schedule for one month assessing quality of life in relation to improvement in functional class using the 6-minute walk test, then each treatment cycle was administered for a period of 8 weeks and symptoms, physical findings and clinical response were re-evaluated. In case of improvement, the treatment cycle was continued at the same interval or reduced accordingly; only in cases of infusion therapy-related symptomatic stability was infusion therapy discontinued for a period of four weeks; after discharge from the cardiac outpatient infusion unit patients were followed up in the congestive heart failure outpatient clinic with twice weekly visits every two weeks monthly at baseline, and then every 2 months.

The study lasted 4 years; during this time stable patients with refractory heart failure symptoms were offered intravenous infusions of inotropes, 18 (25%) patients died, and 6 (8%) patients were withdrawn from the programme by their primary care physician due to significant travel limitations; 4 (5%) patients required continuous intravenous home therapy; and 44 (61%) patients were discharged from the cardiac outpatient infusion unit as a result of significant improvement in their heart failure symptoms. The treatment was well tolerated and no other significant side effects were reported. In total, 1,737 individual outpatient treatment sessions were administered with an average of

24 ± 19 sessions per patient, representing a minimum of 9,948 h of inotropic therapy[11]

.

Baseline and end-of-study values for quality-of-life scores in both patients receiving inotropes and those receiving placebo differed significantly (p<0.001) (fig.4 A). Baseline and end-of-study values for 6-minute walk test scores also differed significantly in the group receiving inotropics (p<0.01), but not in the group receiving placebo (p<0.4)[12] (fig.4 B).

In 2018 a meta-analysis compiled 66 studies of ambulatory inotropic therapy including 13 randomised controlled, 4 non-randomised and 49 observational trials, resulting mostly small with a median of 34.5 cases. The most commonly used drug was dobutamine (74.2% of studies) and administration was intermittent in 50%. The indication was unspecified in 51.5% of the studies, but a combination of bridging and palliative use was represented by 19.7%; individually bridging therapy accounted for 16.7% and palliative use for 12.1% of the total; mortality was 4.2% with no differences between the two indications. There was also no difference between continuous and intermittent use. All-cause hospitalisation was 22.2%, while HF-specific hospitalisation was 10.1%. Before inotropic use, all patients were in CFIII or IV, whereas after use, a 1.2 point reduction in CF was observed[12] .

Many of the studies reviewed concluded that the use of inotropics as palliative therapy could be one of the alternatives that can be offered in professional and family consensus to this group of patients.(Table 2).

3.6.- INOTROPICS MOST COMMONLY USED IN PALLIATIVE THERAPY.

Inotropics are drugs that improve myocardial contractility in situations where pump failure becomes eminent in various clinical scenarios, their indications differ according to the desired outcomes at the time. In the reviews performed, inotropes commonly used as a palliative strategy include milrinone and dobutamine; within the statistical analysis the use of inotropes was variable with dobutamine with an average of 61% more commonly used compared to milrinone with 49% (table 1). The use of these drugs was associated with an improvement in symptoms and a reduction in hospitalisations, levosimendan is also being used as a bridging therapy to transplantation or device, but within its guidelines it indirectly improves quality of life and decreases hospitalisations so it is being analysed as palliative therapy[20] .

The current use of inotropics as palliative therapy is being consolidated within modern strategies to improve the quality of life of patients with end-stage heart failure, but it is not yet established as a protocol due to the lack of consensus building in this area. However, small studies show that it is possible to implement these treatments and that in the future they will be established in cardiovascular care centres, accepting the reality of what this disease implies for the patient in the final phase.

3.7.- DOSAGE OF INOTROPES IN PALLIATIVE CARE.

The analysis of the studies shares in common that inotropic therapy is initiated with the lowest doses of drugs, and titrated according to the haemodynamic response of the patient, there is no standard dose for use in palliative therapy.

The average doses used in the studies analysed in this work were dobutamine with a minimum dose of 2.5 mcg/kg/min and a maximum dose of 4.3 mcg/kg/min; milrinone with a minimum dose of 0.25 mcg/kg/min and a maximum dose of 0.4 mcg/kg/min (Table 4).

3.8.- RISKS AND COMPLICATIONS.

Data on the efficacy of inotropes as palliative therapy compared to conventional medical treatment are limited, and it is essential to communicate the risks and benefits by establishing a patient-physician agreement on the necessary information before starting therapy.

The main complications associated with home inotropic therapy are arrhythmias and infections. In a meta-analysis 41 studies reported that the incidence of ventricular arrhythmias associated with ICD shocks was similar with a range of 2.2 to 3.0 per 100 patients at 1-month follow-up, with a pooled incidence of 2.4 (95% CI 2.1 to 2.8), while 20 studies reported a low rate of sudden death events between 0 to 6 events per study, and given the variability in ICD use between studies the results were not pooled[12].

In a 2016 cohort of 197 patients receiving inotropics for palliative purposes 17% received 1 or more ICD shocks of which[14] were appropriate. The predictor of ICD shocks was reported to be the manifestation of ventricular tachycardia.

Other complications included central line infections; in an analysis of 13 studies, data from 360 patients were collected and pooled, and the rate of central line infection varied by as much as 5-10% in relation to the total number of patients in follow-up for each month[12].

In another study, a group of 197 patients receiving inotropic drugs for different purposes, including palliative treatment which accounted for 29%, infections were reported to be due to puncture site involvement in 10%, bacteraemia without sepsis 70%, endocarditis 5%, sepsis 4%[14].

3.9.- CONTRAINDICATIONS TO INOTROPIC PALLIATIVE THERAPY.

There are underlying conditions that are contraindications to home inotropes, including uncontrolled or refractory arrhythmias and severe outflow tract obstruction, such as aortic or pulmonary stenosis. Severe renal dysfunction is a contraindication for chronic milrinone, but not for dobutamine. Conversely, many inotrope-dependent patients may also require haemodialysis; however, given the overall poor prognosis of these patients the use of inotropes in this population should be considered on a case-by-case basis. In addition, not all dialysis centres admit inotrope-dependent patients. Finally, recent use of additional intravenous drugs is considered to be a relative contraindication for outpatient intravenous inotropics[15].

CHAPTER II
OPERATIONAL APPROACH

METHODOLOGICAL FRAMEWORK.

From the methodological point of view, the research has a quantitative approach, the design and type of research is descriptive. According to the type of research, it is a field study, the technique used is observational, and the temporality is current cross-sectional.

2.-POPULATION AND SAMPLE.

The study population was 336 elderly patients with a mean age of 65 years, with no variability in race, sex and marital status, obtained from the different literature reviews.

2.1.- Selection criteria. The following selection criteria were taken into account for the formalisation of the population:

2.1.a. -Inclusion criteria. The following were included in the present study:

- Articles in which inotropes are used for palliative purposes.
- Literature reviews that include in their study impact on quality of life in patients with CTI associated with inotropic use.

2.1.b-Exclusion criteria. The following were excluded from the study:

- Articles in which inotropes were not used for palliative purposes.
- Studies in which the impact on the quality of life of the study population was not assessed.

3.-OPERATIONALISATION OF VARIABLES

VARIABLE	CONCEPTUAL DEFINITION	OPERATIONAL DEFINITION	INDICATOR	STATISTICAL TYPE	SCALE
Inotropics for palliative purposes.	Drugs that act on myocardial contractility, in patients whose life expectancy is relatively short due to a disease that does not respond to curative treatments	The measurement of inotropics for palliative purposes, taking into account joint professional eligibility guidelines.	Negative Positive	Quantitative	Discreet absence presence
Quality of life	It is an individual's perception of his or her life situation as, in the context of his or her culture and value systems, in relation to his or her goals, expectations,	The measurement was carried out in the 6-minute walk test.	Negative Positive	Quantitative	Discreet. Increase CF Decrease CF

	standards and concerns" are limited.				
End-stage heart failure	Heart failure (HF) is a progressive disorder with high mortality and a heavy symptom burden.	The measurement was carried out in the 6-minute walk test.	Negative Positive	Quantitative	Discreet. Increase CF Decrease CF
Probability of survival	Percentage of people in a study or treatment group who remain alive for a certain period of time after diagnosis or treatment of a disease such as CTI.	It was assessed in terms of time associated with the use of inotropes.	Kaplan Meier survival curve	Quantitative	Discreet. Increase Decrease

Sex	The set of biological, physical, physiological and anatomical characteristics that define human beings as male and female.	The measurement of sex is determined by the information provided.	DNI	Qualitative	Nominal
Age	It is the period in which the life of a living being is spent.	The age measurement is determined by the information provided.	DNI	Qualitative	Nominal

4.- INSTRUMENTS, MATERIALS AND RESOURCES FOR DATA COLLECTION

4.1.- Documentary instruments.

A review was carried out of scientific databases such as PubMed, Medline, Scopus, and Medes, studies related to the use of inotropic drugs for palliative purposes in patients diagnosed with terminal heart failure, including systematic reviews and meta-analyses, taking into account that the intervention was carried out in patients with decompensation due to their own evolution of the disease.

4.2.- Mechanical instruments. A desktop computer, Core I5 processor, was used for data collection.

4.3.- Materials

Desk materials were used.

5.-PROCEDURE FOR DATA COLLECTION

5.1.- Spatial location.

The city of Buenos Aires is located in South America, at 34° 36' south latitude and 58° 26' west longitude, on the banks of the Rio de la Plata.

Just off the coast of Uruguay is Colonia del Sacramento, and further away is Montevideo, the capital of Uruguay, 220 km away (25 min by plane or 2 h 30 by boat). At 1065 km (1 h 50 by plane) is Asunción, the capital of Paraguay; at 1139 km (2 h by plane), Santiago, the capital of Chile; and a little further, at 1719 km (3 h by plane), is São Paulo (Brazil), the other great metropolis of South America.

5.2.-Temporary location.

The research was carried out without distinction of dates.

5.3.- Data collection procedure.

For the recording of data, the following procedure was used:

- Scientific databases such as PubMed, Medline, Scopus, and Medes related studies on the use of inotropics for palliative purposes in patients diagnosed with end-stage heart failure included systematic reviews and meta-analyses.

CHAPTER III
RESULTS, DISCUSSION AND CONCLUSIONS

1. RESULTS

A total of 30 studies that met the inclusion criteria were analysed, varying in design (prospective, n=4; retrospective, n=2, clinical trials=5, reviews=20); the studies collectively included 336 patients, mean age 65 years, with no variability in race, sex and marital status.

All studies assessed quality of life demonstrating improvement in NYHA functional class (decreasing on average 1.5 points). The 6-minute walk test increased by the same percentage as CF. Hospital admissions decreased by 50% since initiation of therapy.

In relation to complications, arrhythmias occurred in 34% of the total patients analysed, and these manifestations were assessed by activation of the ICD. Another complication was catheter-associated infection (central line) in 12% of the patients treated.

The maximum time over which the variables were assessed is related to the duration of therapy for each patient.

Tables of results will be presented:

Table 1. Studies included in the systematic review.

TABLE N°1		
Detail	**Frequency**	**%**
Prospective		13%
Retrospective		7%
Clinical Trials		13%
Systematic Reviews		67%
TOTAL	**30**	**100%**

n Absolute frequency

Relative frequency

Interpretation of the table: In this table it can be seen that 67% of the studies were systematic reviews, while 13% corresponded to Prospective studies, as well as Clinical Trials.

Table 2. Inotropics for palliative purposes.

TABLE 2		
Detail	**Frequency**	**%**
Negative	0	0%
Positive	30	100%
TOTAL	30	100%

n Absolute frequency

Relative frequency

Interpretation of the table: In this table it can be evidenced that 100% of the studies were with inotropics and palliative purposes.

Table 3. Improvement of functional class with the 6 min. walk test.

TABLE N° 3		
Detail	**Frequency**	**%**
Increase	26	87%
Decrease		13%
TOTAL	**30**	**100%**

n Absolute frequency

Relative frequency

Interpretation of the table: In this table it can be seen that 87% showed an improvement in the 6 min bedtime test, while 13% decreased.

Table 4. **Evaluation of studies, End-stage heart failure in relation to hospitalisation treated with Inotropics palliatively.**

TABLE 4		
Detail	**Frequency**	**%**
Decrease		50%
Increase		50%
TOTAL	**30**	**100%**

n Absolute frequency

Relative frequency

Interpretation of the table: This table shows a reduction in hospitalisation in patients treated with inotropic palliative treatment for end-stage heart failure, equivalent to a 50% reduction in the number of hospital admissions.

Table 5. Risk of bias graph: reviewers' judgements of each risk of bias element are presented as percentages across all included studies.

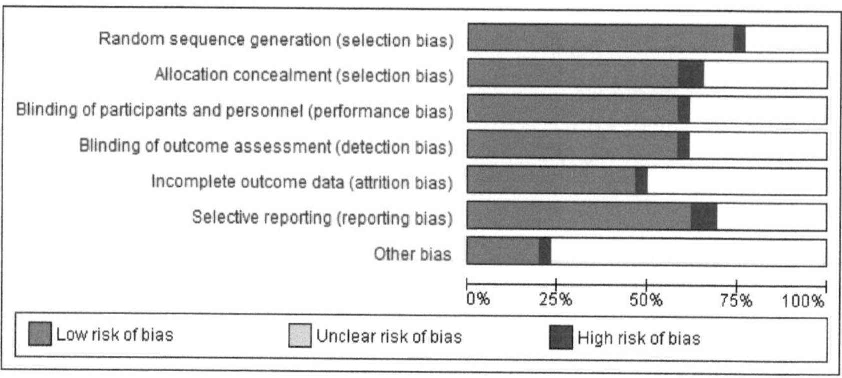

Interpretation of the table: This table shows that most of the studies included in the systematic review had a low risk of bias.

Table 6. Summary of risk of bias: the reviewers' judgements about each element of risk of bias for each included study.

Study	Random sequence generation (selection bias)	Allocation concealment (selection bias)	Blinding of participants and personnel (performance bias)	Blinding of outcome assessment (detection bias)	Incomplete outcome data (attrition bias)	Selective reporting (reporting bias)	Other bias
Angel Lopez 2004	+	+	+	+			
Clyde W. Yancy 2013	+	+		+		+	+
David Cesario 1998	+	+		+		+	+
Dio Kavalieratos 2017	+	+	+		+	+	
Fabrizio Oliva 2018	+		+	+		–	
Francesc Formiga 2019	+	+		+	+	+	
Geetha Bha 2006	+		+	+	+		
Gianfranco Sinagra 2020			+			+	
James B. Young 2000	+	+		+		+	
Jason P. Graffagnino 2020	+		+		+	+	+
Josep Comín-Colet 2018		+		+	+		
Kasey Malotte 2017	+	+		+		+	
Keisuke Kida 2020	+	–	+	+			+
Krishna Pate 2019		+		+	+	+	
Levin RL 2020	+	+	+	+	+	+	
Mahazarin Ginwalla 2016	+		+		+		
Mahazarin Ginwalla 2018			+	+		+	
Michael Taitel 2012		+	+		+	+	+
Mustafa Toma 2010	+		+		+		
Ray E. Hershberger 2003	+		+				
Sara E. Wordingham 2016	+		+			+	
Sarah Chuzi 2019		+		+		+	
Sonja Fruhwald 2016	+	+		+	+	+	
Taimoor Hashim 2015	+	+				+	
Tiana Nizamic 2018	–	–	–	–	–	–	–
William W. Mc Closkey 1998	+	+	+		+		

Interpretation of the table: In this table it can be evidenced that in most of the studies included in the systematic review presented low risk of bias, only one study presented high risk of bias.

2. DISCUSSION

The use of inotropes as palliative therapy in CTI has been described since the 1990s with little evidence, however, there are studies culminating in the recommendations of Clyde W. Yancy (2013) in which he published the AHA inotropic support guidelines.

In the present investigation it was shown that the use of inotropic drugs was determinant in the improvement of CF, the 6-minute walk test, as well as reducing hospital readmission.

This systematic review identified that the quality of data assessing risk/benefit of inotropes is acceptable, taking into consideration the careful interpretation of the results. Most of the studies were small determining diversity in biases and the outpatient inotropic infusion interventions were observational reporting the experience of patients treated with inotropics without a comparison group. Assessment of parameters such as mortality, quality of life, NYHA functional class can be problematic in a population with such a high death rate, often the sickest people are not represented in the follow-up and may contribute to biases.

The study by Lopez et al. analysed 73 patients and concluded that inotropics for outpatient palliative purposes significantly reduced readmission, improved FC and quality of life, with a favourable clinical outcome for most patients.

The main complications are central line infection, high percentage of arrhythmias evidenced by ICDs.

In a 2018 meta-analysis by the group of Tiana Nizamic, MD et al. compared the use of inotropics as a bridge to surgery and as palliative therapy showing that the functional class of the majority of patients in both groups, which was initially III/IV, decreased by 1.2 points. This result contrasts with the data of this review.

3. CONCLUSION

This study was supported by a series of papers with the aim of emphasising inotropic palliative therapy in end-stage heart failure, the analysis of which yielded a positive result in relation to the search for future therapeutic options to improve quality of life in the final phase of the disease.

It was determined in this review that palliative use of inotropes in end-stage heart failure improved CF, quality of life and reduced hospital readmissions.

In terms of risks, the patient was not exempt from complications such as ventricular arrhythmias and infections associated with the central line.

III.- BIBLIOGRAPHY.

1. Formigaa, F. (2007). End-stage heart failure. Med Clin (Barc). 2007;128(7):263-7, 5.

2. Fernando Rodríguez-Artalejo (2004). Epidemiology of heart failure. Rev Esp Cardiol 2004;57(2):163-70, 163-164.

3. Piotr Ponikowski* (Chair) (Poland), Adriaan A. Voors* (2016). ESC 2016 guideline on the diagnosis and treatment of failure. Rev Esp Cardiol. 2016;69(12):1167.e1-e85, e7,3.3.

4. Salim S. Virani, M. (2020). Heart Disease and Stroke Statistics-. Circulation. 2020;, e371.

5. Sinagra, G. (2020). Practical indications for effective implementation of palliative care in patients with heart failure. G Ital Cardiol 2020.

6. Ginwalla, M. M. (2016). Inotropic and other palliative care initiation. . Elsevier , 2.

7. Clyde W. Yancy (2013). 2013 ACCF/AHA Guideline for the. JACC Vol. 62, e191.

8. Sarah Chuzi, M. (2019). Palliative therapy with inotropes. JAMACardiology , E3.

9. Levin RL, R. C. (2020). Consensus on Inotropes and Care. Rev Argent Cardiol 2020.

10. Ray E. Hershberger, M. D. (2003). Care Processes and Clinical Outcomes of Continuous Outpatient Support With Inotropes (COSI) in Patients With Refractory Endstage Heart Failure. Journal of Cardiac Failure Vol. 9 No. 3 2003.

11. Angel Lopez-Candales, M. F. (2004). Need for Hospice and Palliative Care Services in Patients with End-Stage Heart. Clin. Cardiol. 27, 23-28 (2004).

12. Tiana Nizamic, M. u. (2018). Ambulatory inotrope infusions in advanced heart failure. JACC.

13. Sonja Fruhwald, P. P. (2016). Advanced heart failure: an assessment of the potential of levosimendan in this end-stage setting and some related ethical considerations. Published by Informa UK Limited.

14. Deepak Acharya, M. M. (2016). Infections, arrhythmias and hospitalisations with home intravenous inotropic therapy. Elsevier.

15. Mustafa Toma (2010). Inotropic therapy for patients with end-stage heart failure. Springer Science. Business Media, LLC 2010, 409 - 419 DOI 10.1007 /.

16. Keisuke Kida, M. P. (2020). Palliative care in patients with advanced heart failure. Heart Failure Clin 16 (2020) Elsevier.

17. Kasey Malotte (n.d.). Continuous cardiac inotropes in patients with end-stage heart failure: an evolving experience. Journal of pain and symptom management (2017), doi: 10.1016 / j.jpainsymman.2017.09.026.

18. Taimoor Hashim, M. (2015). Clinical characteristics and outcomes of intravenous inotropic therapy in advanced heart failure. circheartfailure.ahajournals DOI: 10.1161/CIRCHEARTFAILURE.114.001778.

19. Patel, K. (2019). Continuous inotropic therapy in palliative care: case series. American Journal of Hospice DOI: 10.1177/1049909118823187.

20. 20. Parle, N. (n.d.). Repeated infusions of levosimendan: well tolerated and improves functional capacity in decompensated heart failure: a single centre experience. Circulation 2008.

21. Oliva, F. (2018). Programmed intermittent inotropics for advanced ambulatory heart failure. Elsevier.

ANNEXES.

Annex 1.

Figure 1. Heart failure.

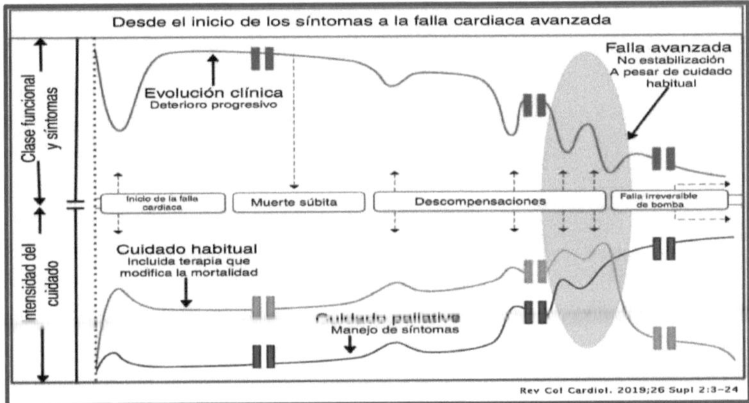

Figure 2 :

Cuestionario sobre la insuficiencia cardiaca (Kansas City) (KCCQ-12)

Las siguientes preguntas se refieren a la **insuficiencia cardiaca** y cómo puede afectar su vida. Por favor, lea y conteste las siguientes preguntas. No hay respuestas correctas ni incorrectas. Por favor, elija la respuesta que corresponda mejor a su situación.

1. La **insuficiencia cardiaca** afecta a las personas de diferentes maneras. Algunas sienten más la falta de aire mientras que otras sienten más la fatiga. Por favor, indique en qué medida la **insuficiencia cardiaca** (por ejemplo, falta de aire o fatiga) ha limitado su capacidad para realizar las siguientes actividades <u>durante las últimas 2 semanas</u>.

Por favor, marque con una **X** un cuadrito en cada línea

Actividad	Extremadamente limitado/a	Bastante limitado/a	Moderadamente limitado/a	Ligeramente limitado/a	Nada limitado/a	Limitado/a por otras razones o no realicé esta actividad
a. Ducharse/bañarse	❑	❑	❑	❑	❑	❑
b. Caminar una cuadra en terreno plano	❑	❑	❑	❑	❑	❑
c. Correr o apresurarse (como para alcanzar el autobús)	❑	❑	❑	❑	❑	❑

2. Durante las <u>últimas 2 semanas</u>, ¿cuántas veces tuvo **hinchazón** de los pies, tobillos o piernas al despertarse en la mañana?

Todas las mañanas	3 o más veces por semana pero no todos los días	1-2 veces por semana	Menos de una vez por semana	Nunca en las últimas 2 semanas
❑	❑	❑	❑	❑

3. Durante las <u>últimas 2 semanas</u>, en promedio, ¿cuántas veces la **fatiga** ha limitado su capacidad para hacer lo que desea?

Todo el tiempo	Varias veces al día	Al menos una vez al día	3 o más veces por semana pero no todos los días	1-2 veces por semana	Menos de una vez por semana	Nunca en las últimas 2 semanas
❑	❑	❑	❑	❑	❑	❑

4. Durante las <u>últimas 2 semanas</u>, en promedio, ¿cuántas veces la **falta de aire** ha limitado su capacidad para hacer lo que desea?

Todo el tiempo	Varias veces al día	Al menos una vez al día	3 o más veces por semana pero no todos los días	1-2 veces por semana	Menos de una vez por semana	Nunca en las últimas 2 semanas
❑	❑	❑	❑	❑	❑	❑

5. Durante las <u>últimas 2 semanas</u>, en promedio, ¿cuántas veces se ha visto obligado/a a dormir sentado/a en un sillón o apoyado/a en por lo menos 3 almohadas al sentir que le **falta el aire**?

Todas las noches	3 o más veces por semana pero no todas las noches	1-2 veces por semana	Menos de una vez por semana	Nunca en las últimas 2 semanas
❑	❑	❑	❑	❑

Copyright ©2012 John Spertus, MD, MPH   KCCQ-12 – Spanish (US)

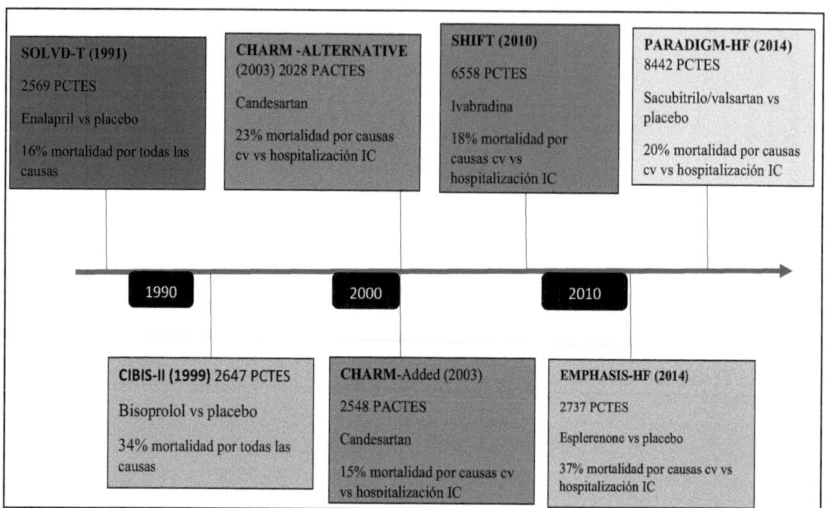

Clinicians

Symptomatic patients who are in stage D HF, refractory to all treatment.

Inotropic dependent with stable dose.

Adequate venous access.

Psychological/Emotional

Understanding the terminal nature of the disease.

Psychological education.

Family and social resources.

Personal health care team: includes nurses trained in the handling of infusion sets and general patient management.

Biosafety available.

Outpatient health follow-up.

TABLE 1: RECOMMENDATIONS FOR INOTROPIC SUPPORT AHA 2013

Recommendations for inotropic support AHA 2013	Level of evidence	Recommendation
Cardiogenic shock pending definitive treatment or resolution A BTT or stage D SCD refractory to conventional treatment.	IIa	B
Short-term support for endangered target organ dysfunction in hospitalised patients with stage D.	IIb	B
Long-term support with continuous infusion palliative therapy in selected stage D HF.	IIb	B
Routine intravenous use, whether continuous or intermittent, is potentially harmful in stage D HF.	III	B
Short-term intravenous use in hospitalised patients without evidence of shock or threatened end-organ function is potentially harmful.	III	B

Annex 2.

Figure 3.1

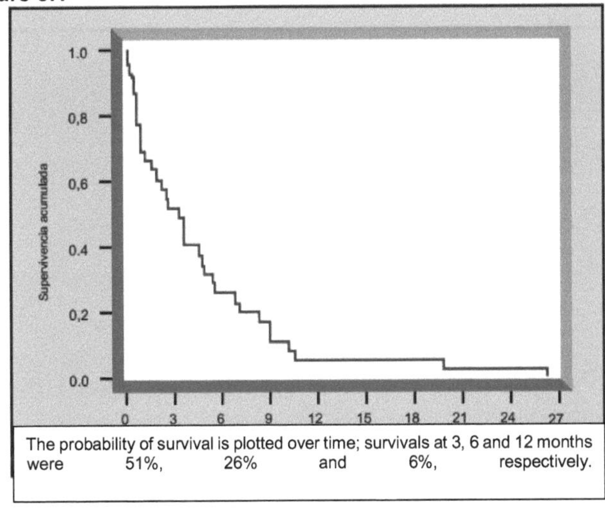

The probability of survival is plotted over time; survivals at 3, 6 and 12 months were 51%, 26% and 6%, respectively.

Figure. 4 A- 4 B

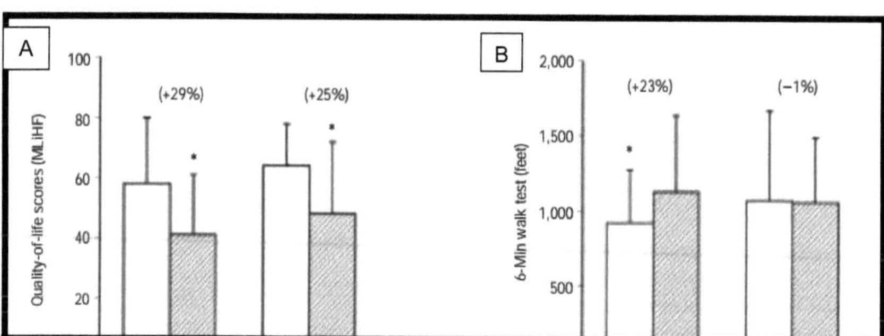

Histogram **A** demonstrating the impact of inotropic drugs on quality of life scores. * Statistically significant difference between baseline and end-of-study values for quality of life scores for patients receiving inotropes (p<0.001) and those receiving placebo (p<0.001).

Histogram **B** demonstrating the impact of inotropic drugs on the results of the 6-minute walk test. * Statistically significant difference between baseline and end-of-study values for 6-minute inotropic gait test results (p<0.01). No difference was found between these values in patients receiving placebo.

Annex 4

Table 2. Specific characteristics of the studies analysed (SR=systematic review, SR=retrospective study, CS=case series)

Kida 2020	RS	13 EA	NA	Palliative	• From the available evidence, inotropic infusions appear to improve **NYHA functional class.** (Keisuke Kida, 2020)
Chuzi 2019	RS	NR	NA	Palliative	• Outpatient inotropic therapy provided symptomatic benefit at the expense of reduced survival, recent data suggest that the survival of patients receiving chronic inotropics may improve over t me.
Patel 2019	ER/SC	NA		Palliative	• Inotropic therapy is being implemented with emphasis and results are favourab e to what is being sought, however, there is little information to support the decision in a general way. (Patel. 2019) (Parle)
Nizamic 2018	RS	66 analysed	NA	Palliative/BTT	• . All-cause hospitalisation was 22.2% per month, while HF-specific hospital sation was 10.1% per month. • A 1.2 point reduction in FC was observed.

Malotte 2017	RS/DC	15 analysed	1 case	Palliative	• Studies analysed showed a reduction in CF by 1 point. • Reduction of hospitalisations in 50% of cases who received inotropics on an outpatient or hospice basis. • Cost comparison in favour of inotropics vs. hospitalisation. (Kasey Malotte)
Fruhwald 2016	RS	Analysed	NA	Palliative	• Analysis of 9 studies with levosimendan and results in favour in terms of reduced hospitalisation and improved biomarkers, positive indicators that could indirectly be met if they are directed towards palliative purposes.
(Taimoor Hashim, 2015)	ER/SC	Randomised trial		Palliative	• Median survival 9.0 months for palliative care patients. • Higher median survival with milrinone • 17% had ≥1 ICD downloads • 29% had ≥1 infections • 57% had ≥1 hospitalisation

Parle 2008	ER	EA		ICA	• 58% were NYHA class IV, mean age 50 (2.4), 82% were male. A significant drop in BNP levels and improvement in NYHA class was observed after infusion.
Lopez 2004	ER/SC	E.OBS		Palliative	• 44 (61%) patients were discharged with significant improvement in their heart failure symptoms.

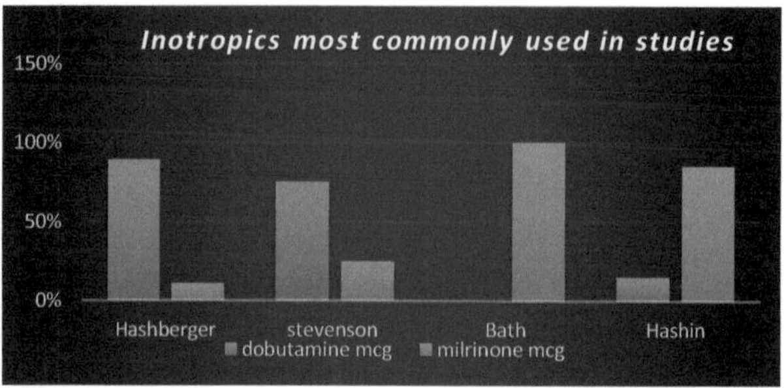
Inotropics most commonly used in studies
150%
100%
50%
0%
Hashberger
stevenson
Bath
Hashin
dobutamine mcg
milrinone mcg

TABLE 3. DIFFERENCES BETWEEN MILRINONE AND DOBUTAMINE

Variable	Milrinona	Dobutamina
Mecanismo de acción	Fosfodiesterasa inhibidor	Agonista β-adrenérgico
Media vida	2 a 4 h	2 minutos
Hemodinámico efectos	HORA ↑, CO ↑, PVR ↓, SVR ↓	HORA ↑↑, CO ↑↑, PVR ↓, SVR ↓↓
Efecto adverso perfil	Arritmogénico, hipotension	Arritmogénico, taquifilaxia periférica eosinofilia, eosinofílica miocarditis
Clínico consideraciones	Reduce PVR, mejor en insuficiencia cardíaca del lado derecho, supervivencia mayor que dobutamina en estudios observacionales	No afectado por la función renal
Costo por mes, $	1000-1400	86-1700
Dosis habitual, rango, µg / kg / min	0,125-0,375	2.5-10

Abreviaturas: CO, gasto cardíaco; FC, frecuencia cardíaca, RVP, resistencia vascular pulmonar; RVS, resistencia vascular sistémica; ↑, incrementar; ↑↑ mayor aumento; ↓, disminuir; ↓↓, mayor disminución.

TABLE. 4

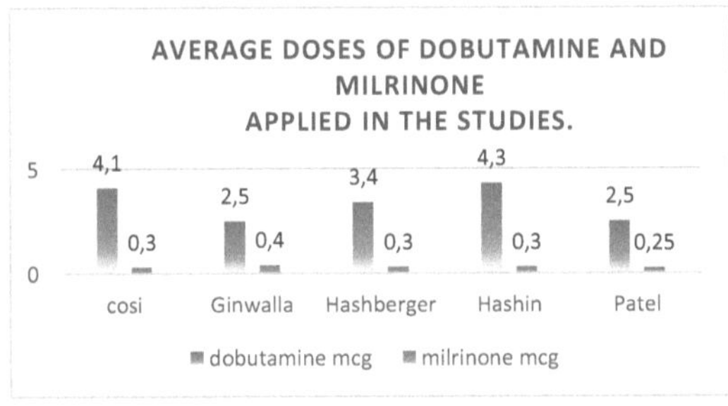

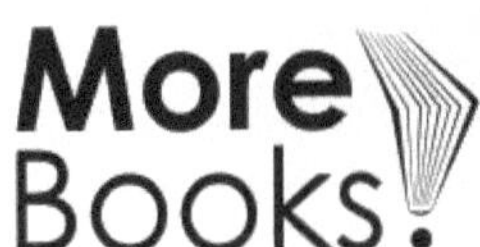

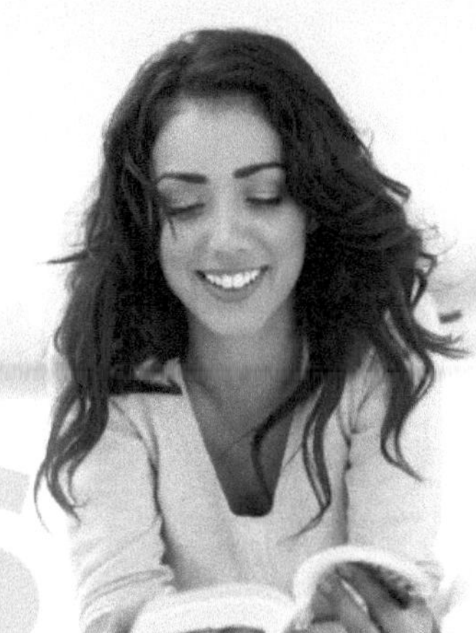

I want morebooks!

Buy your books fast and straightforward online - at one of world's fastest growing online book stores! Environmentally sound due to Print-on-Demand technologies.

Buy your books online at
www.morebooks.shop

Kaufen Sie Ihre Bücher schnell und unkompliziert online – auf einer der am schnellsten wachsenden Buchhandelsplattformen weltweit! Dank Print-On-Demand umwelt- und ressourcenschonend produziert.

Bücher schneller online kaufen
www.morebooks.shop

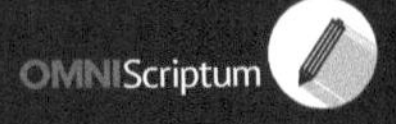

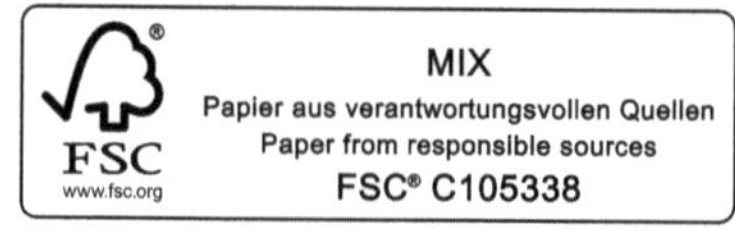

Printed by Books on Demand GmbH, Norderstedt / Germany